Reminiscences of
The Elephant Man

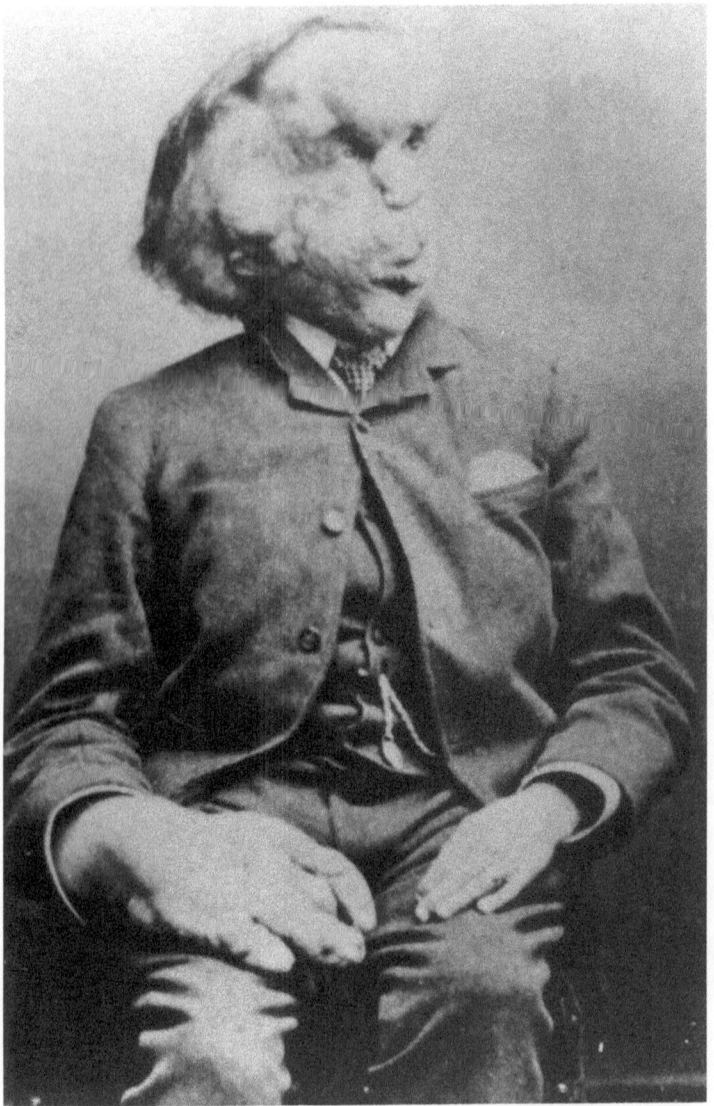

REMINISCENCES OF THE ELEPHANT MAN

by
Sir Frederick Treves
and others

Curious
PUBLICATIONS
New York

Published by Curious Publications
101 W. 23rd St. #318
New York, NY 10011
curiouspublications.com

Copyright © 2021

ISBN-13: 978-1-7353201-1-3

Photo credits:
Cover, frontispiece, pages 8 & 69, Wikimedia Commons; back cover,
pages 64-67, The Wellcome Collection; page 68, Marc Hartzman.

Printed and bound in the United States of America.

A NOTE ON THE TEXT

Tragic as the life of Joseph Merrick was, Sir Frederick Treves' compassion for and friendship with the Elephant Man is to be celebrated. Though the doctor's studies couldn't cure his patient, the time that Treves spent with him revealed a side of Merrick that had been hidden away. The Elephant Man's intellect, joy in the little things, and positive attitude despite his challenges were a triumph of humanity. This text is reprinted from Treves' 1923 book, *The Elephant Man and Other Reminiscences*. The newspaper articles that follow share additional details of Merrick's life and death.

CONTENTS

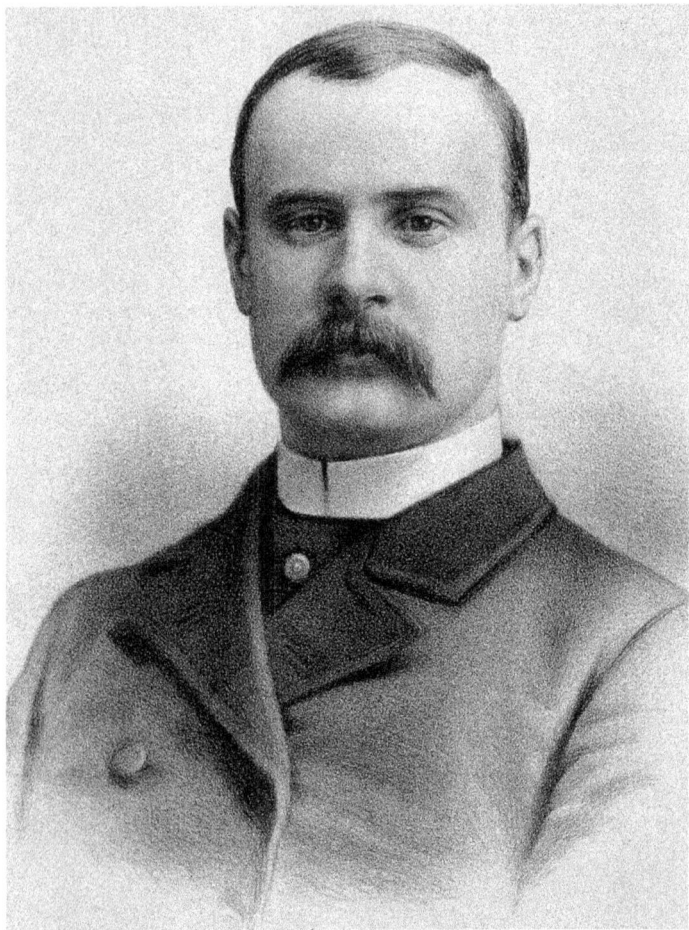

Sir Frederick Treves, 1884.

The Elephant Man

IN THE Mile End Road, opposite to the London Hospital, there was (and possibly still is) a line of small shops. Among them was a vacant greengrocer's which was to let. The whole of the front of the shop, with the exception of the door, was hidden by a hanging sheet of canvas on which was the announcement that the Elephant Man was to be seen within and that the price of admission was twopence. Painted on the canvas in primitive colours was a life-size portrait of the Elephant Man. This very crude production depicted a frightful creature that could only have been possible in a nightmare. It was the figure of a man with the characteristics of an elephant. The transfiguration was not far advanced. There was still more of the man than of the beast. This fact—that it was still human—was the most repellent attribute of the creature. There was nothing about it of the pitiableness of the misshapened or the deformed, nothing of the grotesqueness of the freak, but merely the loathsome insinuation of a man being changed into an animal. Some palm trees in the background of the picture suggested a jungle and might have led the imaginative to assume that it was in this wild that the perverted object had roamed.

When I first became aware of this phenomenon the exhibition was closed, but a well-informed boy sought the proprietor in a public house and I was granted a private view on payment of a shilling. The shop was empty and grey with dust. Some old tins and a few shrivelled potatoes occupied a shelf and some vague vegetable refuse the window. The light in the place was dim, being obscured by the painted placard outside. The far end of the shop—where I expect the late proprietor sat at a desk—was cut off by a curtain or rather by a red tablecloth suspended from a cord by a few rings. The room was cold and dank, for it was the month of November. The year, I might say, was 1884.

The showman pulled back the curtain and re-vealed a bent figure crouching on a stool and covered by a brown blanket. In front of it, on a tripod, was a large brick heated by a Bunsen burner. Over this the creature was huddled to warm itself. It never moved when the curtain was drawn back. Locked up in an empty shop and lit by the faint blue light of the gas jet, this hunched-up figure was the embodiment of loneliness. It might have been a captive in a cavern or a wizard watching for unholy manifestations in the ghostly flame. Outside the sun was shining and one could hear the footsteps of the passers-by, a tune whistled by a boy and the companionable hum of traffic in the road.

The showman—speaking as if to a dog—called out harshly: "Stand up!" The thing arose slowly and let the blanket that covered its head and back fall to the ground. There stood revealed the most disgusting specimen of humanity that I have ever seen. In the course of my profession I had come upon lamentable deformities of the face due to injury or disease, as well as mutilations and contortions of the body depending upon like causes; but at no time had I met with such a degraded or perverted version of a human being as this lone figure displayed. He was naked to the waist, his feet were bare, he wore a pair of threadbare trousers that had once belonged to some fat gentleman's dress suit.

From the intensified painting in the street I had imagined the Elephant Man to be of gigantic size. This, however, was a little man below the average height and made to look shorter by the bowing of his back. The most striking feature about him was his enormous and misshapened head. From the brow there projected a huge bony mass like a loaf, while from the back of the head hung a bag of spongy, fungous-looking skin, the surface of which was comparable to brown cauliflower. On the top of the skull were a few long lank hairs. The osseous growth on the forehead almost occluded one eye. The circumference of the head was no less than that of the man's waist. From the upper jaw there projected another mass of bone. It protruded from the mouth like a pink stump, turning the upper lip inside out and making of the mouth a mere slobbering aperture. This growth from the jaw had been so exaggerated in the painting as to appear to be a rudimentary trunk or tusk. The nose was merely a lump of flesh, only recognizable as a nose from its position. The face was no more capable of expression than a block of gnarled wood. The back was horrible, because from it hung, as far down as the middle of the thigh, huge, sack-like masses of flesh covered by the same loathsome cauliflower skin.

The right arm was of enormous size and shapeless. It suggested the limb of the subject of elephantiasis. It was overgrown also with pendent masses of the same cauliflower-like skin. The hand was large and clumsy—a fin or paddle rather than a hand. There was no distinction between the palm and the back. The thumb had the appearance of a radish, while the fingers might have been thick, tuberous roots. As a limb it was almost useless. The other arm was remarkable by contrast. It was not only normal but was, moreover, a delicately shaped limb covered with fine skin and provided with a beautiful hand which any woman might have envied. From the chest hung a bag of the same repulsive flesh. It was like a dewlap suspended from the neck of a lizard. The lower limbs had the characters of the deformed arm. They were unwieldy, dropsical looking and grossly misshapened.

To add a further burden to his trouble the wretched man, when a boy, developed hip disease, which had left him permanently lame, so that he could only walk with a stick. He was thus denied all means of escape from his tormentors. As he told me later, he could never run away. One other feature must be mentioned to emphasize his isolation from his kind. Although he was already repellent enough, there arose from the fungous skin-growth with which he was almost covered a very sickening stench which was hard to tolerate. From the showman I learnt nothing about the Elephant Man, except that he was English, that his name was John Merrick and that he was twenty-one years of age.

As at the time of my discovery of the Elephant

Man I was the Lecturer on Anatomy at the Medical College opposite, I was anxious to examine him in detail and to prepare an account of his abnormalities. I therefore arranged with the showman that I should interview his strange exhibit in my room at the college. I became at once conscious of a difficulty. The Elephant Man could not show himself in the streets. He would have been mobbed by the crowd and seized by the police. He was, in fact, as secluded from the world as the Man with the Iron Mask. He had, however, a disguise, although it was almost as startling as he was himself. It consisted of a long black cloak which reached to the ground. Whence the cloak had been obtained I cannot imagine. I had only seen such a garment on the stage wrapped about the figure of a Venetian bravo. The recluse was provided with a pair of bag-like slippers in which to hide his deformed feet. On his head was a cap of a kind that never before was seen. It was black like the cloak, had a wide peak, and the general outline of a yachting cap. As the circumference of Merrick's head was that of a man's waist, the size of this headgear may be imagined. From the attachment of the peak a grey flannel curtain hung in front of the face. In this mask was cut a wide horizontal slit through which the wearer could look out. This costume, worn by a bent man hobbling along with a stick, is probably the most remarkable and the most uncanny that has as yet been designed. I arranged that Merrick should cross the road in a cab, and to insure his immediate admission to the college I gave him my card. This card was destined to play a critical part in Merrick's life.

I made a careful examination of my visitor the result of which I embodied in a paper.[1] I made little of the man himself. He was shy, confused, not a little frightened and evidently much cowed. Moreover, his speech was almost unintelligible. The great bony mass that projected from his mouth blurred his utterance and made the articulation of certain words impossible. He returned in a cab to the place of exhibition, and I assumed that I had seen the last of him, especially as I found next day that the show had been forbidden by the police and that the shop was empty.

I supposed that Merrick was imbecile and had been imbecile from birth. The fact that his face was incapable of expression, that his speech was a mere spluttering and his attitude that of one whose mind was void of all emotions and concerns gave grounds for this belief. The conviction was no doubt encouraged by the hope that his intellect was the

---

1 *British Medical Journal*, Dec., 1886, and April, 1890.

blank I imagined it to be. That he could appreci-
ate his position was unthinkable. Here was a man
in the heyday of youth who was so vilely deformed
that everyone he met confronted him with a look of
horror and disgust. He was taken about the country
to be exhibited as a monstrosity and an object of
loathing. He was shunned like a leper, housed like a
wild beast, and got his only view of the world from
a peephole in a showman's cart. He was, moreover,
lame, had but one available arm, and could hardly
make his utterances understood. It was not until I
came to know that Merrick was highly intelligent,
that he possessed an acute sensibility and—worse
than all—a romantic imagination that I realized the
overwhelming tragedy of his life.

The episode of the Elephant Man was, I imagined, closed; but I was fated to meet him again—
two years later—under more dramatic conditions.
In England the showman and Merrick had been
moved on from place to place by the police, who
considered the exhibition degrading and among
the things that could not be allowed. It was hoped
that in the uncritical retreats of Mile End a more
abiding peace would be found. But it was not to be.
The official mind there, as elsewhere, very properly
decreed that the public exposure of Merrick and his
deformities transgressed the limits of decency. The

show must close.

The showman, in despair, fled with his charge to the Continent. Whither he roamed at first I do not know; but he came finally to Brussels. His reception was discouraging. Brussels was firm; the exhibition was banned; it was brutal, indecent and immoral, and could not be permitted within the confines of Belgium. Merrick was thus no longer of value. He was no longer a source of profitable entertainment. He was a burden. He must be got rid of. The elimination of Merrick was a simple matter. He could offer no resistance. He was as docile as a sick sheep. The impresario, having robbed Merrick of his paltry savings, gave him a ticket to London, saw him into the train and no doubt in parting condemned him to perdition.

His destination was Liverpool Street. The journey may be imagined. Merrick was in his alarming outdoor garb. He would be harried by an eager mob as he hobbled along the quay. They would run ahead to get a look at him. They would lift the hem of his cloak to peep at his body. He would try to hide in the train or in some dark corner of the boat, but never could he be free from that ring of curious eyes or from those whispers of fright and aversion. He had but a few shillings in his pocket and nothing either to eat or drink on the way. A panic-dazed dog with a label on his collar would have received some sympathy and possibly some kindness. Merrick received none.

What was he to do when he reached London? He had not a friend in the world. He knew no more of London than he knew of Pekin. How could he find a lodging, or what lodging-house keeper would dream of taking him in? All he wanted was to hide. What most he dreaded were the open street and the gaze of his fellow-men. If even he crept into a cellar the horrid eyes and the still more dreaded whispers would follow him to its depths. Was there ever such a homecoming!

At Liverpool Street he was rescued from the crowd by the police and taken into the third-class waiting-room. Here he sank on the floor in the darkest corner. The police were at a loss what to do with him. They had dealt with strange and mouldy tramps, but never with such an object as this. He could not explain himself. His speech was so maimed that he might as well have spoken in Arabic. He had, however, something with him which he produced with a ray of hope. It was my card.

The card simplified matters. It made it evident that this curious creature had an acquaintance and that the individual must be sent for. A messenger was dispatched to the London Hospital which is comparatively near at hand. Fortunately I was in the building and returned at once with the messenger to the station. In the waiting-room I had some difficulty in making a way through the crowd, but there, on the floor in the corner, was Merrick. He looked a mere heap. It seemed as if he had been thrown there like a bundle. He was so huddled up and so helpless looking that he might have had both his arms and his legs broken. He seemed pleased to see me, but he was nearly done. The journey and want of food had reduced him to the last stage of exhaustion. The police kindly helped him into a cab, and I drove him at once to the hospital. He appeared to be content, for he fell asleep almost as soon as he was seated and slept to the journey's end. He never said a word, but seemed to be satisfied that all was well.

In the attics of the hospital was an isolation ward with a single bed. It was used for emergency purposes—for a case of delirium tremens, for a man who had become suddenly insane or for a patient with an undetermined fever. Here the Elephant Man was deposited on a bed, was made comfortable and was supplied with food. I had been guilty of an irregularity in admitting such a case, for the hospital was neither a refuge nor a home for incurables. Chronic cases were not accepted, but only those requiring active treatment, and Merrick was not in need of such treatment. I applied to the sympathetic chairman of the committee, Mr. Carr Gomm, who not only was good enough to approve my action but who agreed with me that Merrick must not again be turned out into the world.

Mr. Carr Gomm wrote a letter to the *Times* detailing the circumstances of the refugee and asking for money for his support. So generous is the English public that in a few days—I think in a week—enough money was forthcoming to maintain Merrick for life without any charge upon the hospital funds. There chanced to be two empty rooms at the back of the hospital which were little used. They were on the ground floor, were out of the way, and opened upon a large courtyard called Bedstead Square, because here the iron beds were marshalled for cleaning and painting. The front room was converted into a bed-sitting room and the smaller chamber into a bathroom. The condition of Merrick's skin rendered a bath at least once a day a necessity, and I might here mention that with the use of the bath the unpleasant odour to which I have referred ceased to be noticeable. Merrick took up his abode in the hospital in December, 1886.

Merrick had now something he had never dreamed of, never supposed to be possible—a home of his own for life. I at once began to make myself acquainted with him and to endeavour to under-stand his mentality. It was a study of much interest. I very soon learnt his speech so that I could talk freely with him. This afforded him great satisfaction, for, curiously enough, he had a passion for conversation, yet all his life had had no one to talk to. I—having then much leisure—saw him almost every day, and made a point of spending some two hours with him every Sunday morning when he would chatter al-most without ceasing. It was unreasonable to expect one nurse to attend to him continuously, but there was no lack of temporary volunteers. As they did not all acquire his speech it came about that I had occasionally to act as an interpreter.

I found Merrick, as I have said, remarkably in-telligent. He had learnt to read and had become a most voracious reader. I think he had been taught when he was in hospital with his diseased hip. His range of books was limited. The Bible and Prayer Book he knew intimately, but he had subsisted for the most part upon newspapers, or rather upon such fragments of old journals as he had chanced to pick up. He had read a few stories and some elementa-ry lesson books, but the delight of his life was a ro-mance, especially a love romance. These tales were very real to him, as real as any narrative in the Bible, so that he would tell them to me as incidents in the lives of people who had lived. In his outlook upon the world he was a child, yet a child with some of the tempestuous feelings of a man. He was an elemental being, so primitive that he might have spent the twenty-three years of his life immured in a cave.

Of his early days I could learn but little. He was very loath to talk about the past. It was a nightmare, the shudder of which was still upon him. He was born, he believed, in or about Leicester. Of his father he knew absolutely nothing. Of his mother he had some memory. It was very faint and had, I think, been elaborated in his mind into something definite. Mothers figured in the tales he had read, and he wanted his mother to be one of those comfortable lullaby-singing persons who are so lovable. In his subconscious mind there was apparently a germ of recollection in which someone figured who had been kind to him. He clung to this conception and made it more real by invention, for since the day when he could toddle no one had been kind to him. As an infant he must have been repellent, although his deformities did not become gross until he had attained his full stature.

It was a favourite belief of his that his mother was beautiful. The fiction was, I am aware, one of his own making, but it was a great joy to him. His mother, lovely as she may have been, basely deserted him when he was very small, so small that his earliest clear memories were of the workhouse to which he had been taken. Worthless and inhuman as this mother was, he spoke of her with pride and even with reverence. Once, when referring to his own appearance, he said: "It *is* very strange, for, you see, mother was so beautiful."

The rest of Merrick's life up to the time that I met him at Liverpool Street Station was one dull record of degradation and squalor. He was dragged from town to town and from fair to fair as if he were a strange beast in a cage. A dozen times a day he would have to expose his nakedness and his piteous deformities before a gaping crowd who greeted him with such mutterings as "Oh! what a horror! What a beast!" He had had no childhood. He had had no boyhood. He had never experienced pleasure. He knew nothing of the joy of living nor of the fun of things. His sole idea of happiness was to creep into the dark and hide. Shut up alone in a booth, awaiting the next exhibition, how mocking must have sounded the laughter and merriment of the boys and girls outside who were enjoying the "fun of the fair"! He had no past to look back upon and no future to look forward to. At the age of twenty he was a creature without hope. There was nothing in front of him but a vista of caravans creeping along a road, of rows of glaring show tents and of circles of staring eyes with, at the end, the spectacle of a broken man in a poor law infirmary.

Those who are interested in the evolution of character might speculate as to the effect of this brutish life upon a sensitive and intelligent man. It would be reasonable to surmise that he would become a spiteful and malignant misanthrope, swollen with venom and filled with hatred of his fellow-men, or, on the other hand, that he would degenerate into a despairing melancholic on the verge of idiocy. Merrick, however, was no such being. He had passed through the fire and had come out unscathed. His troubles had ennobled him. He showed himself to be a gentle, affectionate and lovable creature, as amiable as a happy woman, free from any trace of cynicism or resentment, without a grievance and without an unkind word for anyone. I have never heard him complain. I have never heard him deplore his ruined life or resent the treatment he had received at the hands of callous keepers. His journey through life had been indeed along a *via dolorosa*, the road had been uphill all the way, and now, when the night was at its blackest and the way most steep, he had suddenly found himself, as it were, in a friendly inn, bright with light and warm with welcome. His gratitude to those about him was pathetic in its sincerity and eloquent in the childlike simplicity with which it was expressed.

As I learnt more of this primitive creature I found that there were two anxieties which were prominent in his mind and which he revealed to me with diffidence. He was in the occupation of the rooms assigned to him and had been assured that he would be cared for to the end of his days. This, however, he found hard to realize, for he often asked me timidly to what place he would next be moved. To understand his attitude it is necessary to remember that he had been moving on and moving on all his life. He knew no other state of existence. To him it was normal. He had passed from the workhouse to the hospital, from the hospital back to the workhouse, then from this town to that town or from one showman's caravan to another. He had never known a home nor any semblance of one. He had no possessions. His sole belongings, besides his clothes and some books, were the monstrous cap and the cloak. He was a wanderer, a pariah and an outcast. That his quarters at the hospital were his for life he could not understand. He could not rid his mind of the anxiety which had pursued him for so many years— where am I to be taken next?

Another trouble was his dread of his fellow-men, his fear of people's eyes, the dread of be-

ing always stared at, the lash of the cruel mutterings of the crowd. In his home in Bedstead Square
he was secluded; but now and then a thoughtless
porter or a wardmaid would open his door to let
curious friends have a peep at the Elephant Man. It
therefore seemed to him as if the gaze of the world
followed him still.

Influenced by these two obsessions he became,
during his first few weeks at the hospital, curiously
uneasy. At last, with much hesitation, he said to me
one day: "When I am next moved can I go to a blind
asylum or to a lighthouse?" He had read about blind
asylums in the newspapers and was attracted by the
thought of being among people who could not see.
The lighthouse had another charm. It meant seclusion from the curious. There at least no one could
open a door and peep in at him. There he would
forget that he had once been the Elephant Man.
There he would escape the vampire showman. He
had never seen a lighthouse, but he had come upon
a picture of the Eddystone, and it appeared to him
that this lonely column of stone in the waste of the
sea was such a home as he had longed for.

I had no great difficulty in ridding Merrick's
mind of these ideas. I wanted him to get accustomed
to his fellow-men, to become a human being himself
and to be admitted to the communion of his kind.

He appeared day by day less frightened, less haunted looking, less anxious to hide, less alarmed when he saw his door being opened. He got to know most of the people about the place, to be accustomed to their comings and goings, and to realize that they took no more than a friendly notice of him. He could only go out after dark, and on fine nights ventured to take a walk in Bedstead Square clad in his black cloak and his cap. His greatest adventure was on one moonless evening when he walked alone as far as the hospital garden and back again.

To secure Merrick's recovery and to bring him, as it were, to life once more, it was necessary that he should make the acquaintance of men and women who would treat him as a normal and intelligent young man and not as a monster of deformity. Women I felt to be more important than men in bringing about his transformation. Women were the more frightened of him, the more disgusted at his appearance and the more apt to give way to irrepressible expressions of aversion when they came into his presence. Moreover, Merrick had an admiration of women of such a kind that it attained almost to adoration. This was not the outcome of his personal experience. They were not real women but the products of his imagination. Among them was the beautiful mother surrounded, at a respectful distance, by heroines from the many romances he had read.

His first entry to the hospital was attended by a regrettable incident. He had been placed on the bed in the little attic, and a nurse had been instructed to bring him some food. Unfortunately she had not been fully informed of Merrick's unusual appearance. As she entered the room she saw on the bed, propped up by white pillows, a monstrous figure as hideous as an Indian idol. She at once dropped the tray she was carrying and fled, with a shriek, through the door. Merrick was too weak to notice much, but the experience, I am afraid, was not new to him.

He was looked after by volunteer nurses whose ministrations were somewhat formal and constrained. Merrick, no doubt, was conscious that their service was purely official, that they were merely doing what they were told to do and that they were acting rather as automata than as women. They did not help him to feel that he was of their kind. On the contrary they, without knowing it, made him aware that the gulf of separation was immeasurable.

Feeling this, I asked a friend of mine, a young and pretty widow, if she thought she could enter Merrick's room with a smile, wish him good morning and shake him by the hand. She said she could and she did. The effect upon poor Merrick was not quite what I had expected. As he let go her hand he bent his head on his knees and sobbed until I thought he would never cease. The interview was over. He told me afterwards that this was the first woman who had ever smiled at him, and the first woman, in the whole of his life, who had shaken hands with him. From this day the transformation of Merrick commenced and he began to change, little by little, from a hunted thing into a man. It was a wonderful change to witness and one that never ceased to fascinate me.

Merrick's case attracted much attention in the papers, with the result that he had a constant succession of visitors. Everybody wanted to see him. He must have been visited by almost every lady of note in the social world. They were all good enough to welcome him with a smile and to shake hands with him. The Merrick whom I had found shivering behind a rag of a curtain in an empty shop was now conversant with duchesses and countesses and other ladies of high degree. They brought him presents, made his room bright with ornaments and pictures, and, what pleased him more than all, supplied him with books. He soon had a large library and most of his day was spent in reading. He was not the least spoiled; not the least puffed up; he never asked for anything; never presumed upon the kindness meted out to him, and was always humbly and profoundly grateful. Above all he lost his shyness. He liked to see his door pushed open and people to look in. He became acquainted with most of the frequenters of Bedstead Square, would chat with them at his window and show them some of his choicest presents. He improved in his speech, although to the end his utterances were not easy for strangers to understand. He was beginning, moreover, to be less conscious of his unsightliness, a little disposed to think it was, after all, not so very extreme. Possibly this was aided by the circumstance that I would not allow a mirror of any kind in his room.

The height of his social development was reached on an eventful day when Queen Alexandra—then Princess of Wales—came to the hospital to pay him a special visit. With that kindness which has marked every act of her life, the Queen entered Merrick's room smiling and shook him warmly by the hand. Merrick was transported with delight. This was beyond even his most extravagant dream. The Queen has made many people happy, but I think no gracious act of hers has ever caused such happiness as she brought into Merrick's room when she sat by his chair and talked to him as to a person she was glad to see.

Merrick, I may say, was now one of the most contented creatures I have chanced to meet. More than once he said to me: "I am happy every hour of the day." This was good to think upon when I recalled the half-dead heap of miserable humanity I had seen in the corner of the waiting-room at Liverpool Street. Most men of Merrick's age would have expressed their joy and sense of contentment by singing or whistling when they were alone. Unfortunately poor Merrick's mouth was so deformed that he could neither whistle nor sing. He was satisfied to express himself by beating time upon the pillow to some tune that was ringing in his head. I have many times found him so occupied when I have entered his room unexpectedly. One thing that always struck me as sad about Merrick was the fact that he could not smile. Whatever his delight might be, his face remained expressionless. He could weep but he could not smile.

The Queen paid Merrick many visits and sent him every year a Christmas card with a message in her own handwriting. On one occasion she sent him a signed photograph of herself. Merrick, quite overcome, regarded it as a sacred object and would hardly allow me to touch it. He cried over it, and after it was framed had it put up in his room as a kind

of ikon. I told him that he must write to Her Royal
Highness to thank her for her goodness. This he was
pleased to do, as he was very fond of writing letters,
never before in his life having had anyone to write
to. I allowed the letter to be dispatched unedited. It
began "My dear Princess" and ended "Yours very
sincerely." Unorthodox as it was it was expressed in
terms any courtier would have envied.

Other ladies followed the Queen's gracious ex-
ample and sent their photographs to this delighted
creature who had been all his life despised and re-
jected of men. His mantelpiece and table became so
covered with photographs of handsome ladies, with
dainty knicknacks and pretty trifles that they may
almost have befitted the apartment of an Adonis-
like actor or of a famous tenor.

Through all these bewildering incidents and
through the glamour of this great change Merrick
still remained in many ways a mere child. He had all
the invention of an imaginative boy or girl, the same
love of "make-believe," the same instinct of "dress-
ing up" and of personating heroic and impressive
characters. This attitude of mind was illustrated by
the following incident. Benevolent visitors had given
me, from time to time, sums of money to be expend-
ed for the comfort of the *ci-devant* Elephant Man.
When one Christmas was approaching I asked Mer-

rick what he would like me to purchase as a Christmas present. He rather startled me by saying shyly that he would like a dressing-bag with silver fittings. He had seen a picture of such an article in an advertisement which he had furtively preserved.

The association of a silver-fitted dressing-bag with the poor wretch wrapped up in a dirty blanket in an empty shop was hard to comprehend. I fathomed the mystery in time, for Merrick made little secret of the fancies that haunted his boyish brain. Just as a small girl with a tinsel coronet and a window curtain for a train will realize the conception of a countess on her way to court, so Merrick loved to imagine himself a dandy and a young man about town. Mentally, no doubt, he had frequently "dressed up" for the part. He could "make-believe" with great effect, but he wanted something to render his fancied character more realistic. Hence the jaunty bag which was to assume the function of the toy coronet and the window curtain that could transform a mite with a pigtail into a countess.

As a theatrical "property" the dressing-bag was ingenious, since there was little else to give substance to the transformation. Merrick could not wear the silk hat of the dandy nor, indeed, any kind of hat. He could not adapt his body to the trimly cut coat. His deformity was such that he could wear neither collar nor tie, while in association with his bulbous feet the young blood's patent leather shoe was unthinkable. What was there left to make up the character? A lady had given him a ring to wear on his undeformed hand, and a noble lord had presented him with a very stylish walking-stick. But these things, helpful as they were, were hardly sufficing.

The dressing-bag, however, was distinctive, was explanatory and entirely characteristic. So the bag was obtained and Merrick the Elephant Man became, in the seclusion of his chamber, the Piccadilly exquisite, the young spark, the gallant, the "nut." When I purchased the article I realized that as Merrick could never travel he could hardly want a dressing-bag. He could not use the silver-backed brushes and the comb because he had no hair to brush. The ivory-handled razors were useless because he could not shave. The deformity of his mouth rendered an ordinary toothbrush of no avail, and as his monstrous lips could not hold a cigarette the cigarette-case was a mockery. The silver shoe-horn would be of no service in the putting on of his ungainly slippers, while the hat-brush was quite unsuited to the peaked cap with its visor.

Still the bag was an emblem of the real swell and of the knockabout Don Juan of whom he had read. So every day Merrick laid out upon his table, with proud precision, the silver brushes, the razors, the shoe-horn and the silver cigarette-case which I had taken care to fill with cigarettes. The contemplation of these gave him great pleasure, and such is the power of self-deception that they convinced him he was the "real thing."

I think there was just one shadow in Merrick's life. As I have already said, he had a lively imagination; he was romantic; he cherished an emotional regard for women and his favourite pursuit was the reading of love stories. He fell in love—in a humble and devotional way—with, I think, every attractive lady he saw. He, no doubt, pictured himself the hero of many a passionate incident. His bodily deformity had left unmarred the instincts and feelings of his years. He was amorous. He would like to have been a lover, to have walked with the beloved object in the languorous shades of some beautiful garden and to have poured into her ear all the glowing utterances that he had rehearsed in his heart. And yet—the pity of it!—imagine the feelings of such a youth when he saw nothing but a look of horror creep over the face of every girl whose eyes met his. I fancy when he talked of life among the blind there was a half-formed idea in his mind that he might be able to win the affection of a woman if only she were without eyes to see.

As Merrick developed he began to display certain modest ambitions in the direction of improving his mind and enlarging his knowledge of the world. He was as curious as a child and as eager to learn. There were so many things he wanted to know and to see. In the first place he was anxious to view the interior of what he called "a real house," such a house as figured in many of the tales he knew, a house with a hall, a drawing-room where guests were received and a dining-room with plate on the sideboard and with easy chairs into which the hero could "fling himself." The workhouse, the common lodging-house and a variety of mean garrets were all the residences he knew. To satisfy this wish I drove him up to my small house in Wimpole Street. He was absurdly interested, and examined everything in detail and with untiring curiosity. I could not show him the pampered menials and the powdered footmen of whom he had read, nor could I produce the white marble staircase of the mansion of romance nor the gilded mirrors and the brocaded divans which belong to that style of residence. I explained that the house was a modest dwelling of the Jane Austen type, and as he had read "Emma" he was content.

A more burning ambition of his was to go to the theatre. It was a project very difficult to satisfy. A popular pantomime was then in progress at Drury Lane Theatre, but the problem was how so conspicuous a being as the Elephant Man could be got there, and how he was to see the performance without attracting the notice of the audience and causing a panic or, at least, an unpleasant diversion. The whole matter was most ingeniously carried through by that kindest of women and most able of actresses—Mrs. Kendal. She made the necessary arrangements with the lessee of the theatre. A box was obtained. Merrick was brought up in a carriage with drawn blinds and was allowed to make use of the royal entrance so as to reach the box by a private stair. I had begged three of the hospital sisters to don evening dress and to sit in the front row in order to "dress" the box, on the one hand, and to form a screen for Merrick on the other. Merrick and I occupied the back of the box which was kept in shadow. All went well, and no one saw a figure, more monstrous than any on the stage, mount the staircase or cross the corridor.

One has often witnessed the unconstrained delight of a child at its first pantomime, but Merrick's rapture was much more intense as well as much more solemn. Here was a being with the brain of a man, the fancies of a youth and the imagination of a child. His attitude was not so much that of delight as of wonder and amazement. He was awed. He was enthralled. The spectacle left him speechless, so that if he were spoken to he took no heed. He often seemed to be panting for breath. I could not help comparing him with a man of his own age in the stalls. This satiated individual was bored to distraction, would look wearily at the stage from time to time and then yawn as if he had not slept for nights; while at the same time Merrick was thrilled by a vision that was almost beyond his comprehension. Merrick talked of this pantomime for weeks and weeks. To him, as to a child with the faculty of make-believe, everything was real; the palace was the home of kings, the princess was of royal blood, the fairies were as undoubted as the children in the street, while the dishes at the banquet were of unquestionable gold. He did not like to discuss it as a play but rather as a vision of some actual world. When this mood possessed him he would say: "I wonder what the prince did after we left," or "Do you think that poor man is still in the dungeon?" and so on and so on.

The splendour and display impressed him, but, I think, the ladies of the ballet took a still greater hold upon his fancy. He did not like the ogres and the giants, while the funny men impressed him as irreverent. Having no experience as a boy of romping and ragging, of practical jokes or of "larks," he had little sympathy with the doings of the clown, but, I think (moved by some mischievous instinct in his subconscious mind), he was pleased when the policeman was smacked in the face, knocked down and generally rendered undignified.

Later on another longing stirred the depths of Merrick's mind. It was a desire to see the country, a desire to live in some green secluded spot and there learn something about flowers and the ways of animals and birds. The country as viewed from a wagon on a dusty high road was all the country he knew. He had never wandered among the fields nor followed the windings of a wood. He had never climbed to the brow of a breezy down. He had never gathered flowers in a meadow. Since so much of his reading dealt with country life he was possessed by the wish to see the wonders of that life himself.

This involved a difficulty greater than that presented by a visit to the theatre. The project was, however, made possible on this occasion also by the kindness and generosity of a lady—Lady Knightley—who offered Merrick a holiday home in a cottage on her estate. Merrick was conveyed to the railway station in the usual way, but as he could hardly venture to appear on the platform the railway authorities were good enough to run a second-class carriage into a distant siding. To this point Merrick was driven and was placed in the carriage unobserved. The carriage, with the curtains drawn, was then attached to the mainline train.

He duly arrived at the cottage, but the housewife (like the nurse at the hospital) had not been made clearly aware of the unfortunate man's appearance. Thus it happened that when Merrick presented himself his hostess, throwing her apron over her head, fled, gasping, to the fields. She affirmed that such a guest was beyond her powers of endurance, for, when she saw him, she was "that took" as to be in danger of being permanently "all of a tremble."

Merrick was then conveyed to a gamekeeper's cottage which was hidden from view and was close to the margin of a wood. The man and his wife were able to tolerate his presence. They treated him with the greatest kindness, and with them he spent the one supreme holiday of his life. He could roam where he pleased. He met no one on his wanderings, for the wood was preserved and denied to all but the gamekeeper and the forester.

There is no doubt that Merrick passed in this retreat the happiest time he had as yet experienced. He was alone in a land of wonders. The breath of the country passed over him like a healing wind.

Into the silence of the wood the fearsome voice of the showman could never penetrate. No cruel eyes could peep at him through the friendly undergrowth. It seemed as if in this place of peace all stain had been wiped away from his sullied past. The Merrick who had once crouched terrified in the filthy shadows of a Mile End shop was now sitting in the sun, in a clearing among the trees, arranging a bunch of violets he had gathered.

His letters to me were the letters of a delighted and enthusiastic child. He gave an account of his trivial adventures, of the amazing things he had seen, and of the beautiful sounds he had heard. He had met with strange birds, had startled a hare from her form, had made friends with a fierce dog, and had watched the trout darting in a stream. He sent me some of the wild flowers he had picked. They were of the commonest and most familiar kind, but they were evidently regarded by him as rare and precious specimens.

He came back to London, to his quarters in Bedstead Square, much improved in health, pleased to be "home" again and to be once more among his books, his treasures and his many friends.

Some six months after Merrick's return from the country he was found dead in bed. This was in April, 1890. He was lying on his back as if asleep, and had evidently died suddenly and without a struggle, since not even the coverlet of the bed was disturbed. The method of his death was peculiar. So large and so heavy was his head that he could not sleep lying down. When he assumed the recumbent position the massive skull was inclined to drop backwards, with the result that he experienced no little distress. The attitude he was compelled to assume when he slept was very strange. He sat up in bed with his back supported by pillows, his knees were drawn up, and his arms clasped round his legs, while his head rested on the points of his bent knees.

He often said to me that he wished he could lie down to sleep "like other people." I think on this last night he must, with some determination, have made the experiment. The pillow was soft, and the head, when placed on it, must have fallen backwards and caused a dislocation of the neck. Thus it came about that his death was due to the desire that had dominated his life—the pathetic but hopeless desire to be "like other people."

As a specimen of humanity, Merrick was ignoble and repulsive; but the spirit of Merrick, if it could be seen in the form of the living, would assume the figure of an upstanding and heroic man, smooth browed and clean of limb, and with eyes that flashed undaunted courage.

His tortured journey had come to an end. All the way he, like another, had borne on his back a burden almost too grievous to bear. He had been plunged into the Slough of Despond, but with manly steps had gained the farther shore. He had been made "a spectacle to all men" in the heartless streets of Vanity Fair. He had been ill-treated and reviled and bespattered with the mud of Disdain. He had escaped the clutches of the Giant Despair, and at last had reached the "Place of Deliverance," where "his burden loosed from off his shoulders and fell from off his back, so that he saw it no more."

THE LIFE AND ADVENTURES OF JOSEPH CAREY MERRICK

A pamphlet allegedly written by Joseph Merrick and sold at exhibitions, prior to being taken in by Sir Frederick Treves.

THE LIFE AND ADVENTURES

JOSEPH CAREY MERRICK,

THE GREAT FREAK OF NATURE!

THE GREAT FREAK OF NATURE!

Half a Man & Half an Elephant.

I first saw the light on the 5th of August, 1860, I was born in Lee Street, Wharf Street, Leicester. The deformity which I am now exhibiting was caused by my mother being frightened by an Elephant; my mother was going along the street when a procession of Animals were passing by, there was a terrible crush of people to see them, and unfortunately she was pushed under the Elephant's feet, which frightened her very much; this occurring during a time of pregnancy was the cause of my deformity.

The measurement around my head is 36 inches, there is a large substance of flesh at the back as large as a breakfast cup, the other part in a manner of speaking is like hills and valleys, all lumped together, while the face is such a sight that no one could describe it. The right hand is almost the size and shape of an Elephant's foreleg, measuring 12 inches round the wrist and 5 inches round one of the fingers; the other hand and arm is no larger than that of a girl ten years of age, although it is well proportioned. My feet and legs are covered with thick lumpy skin, also my body, like that of an Elephant, and almost the same colour, in fact, no one would believe until they saw it, that such a thing could exist. It was not perceived much at birth, but began to develop itself when at the age of 5 years.

I went to school like other children until I was about 11 or 12 years of age, when the greatest misfortune of my life occurred, namely—the death of my mother, peace to her, she was a good mother to me; after she died my father broke up his home and went to lodgings; unfortunately for me he married his landlady; henceforth I never had one moment's comfort, she having children of her own, and I not being so handsome as they, together with my deformity, she was the means of making my life a perfect misery; lame and deformed as I was, I ran, or rather walked away from home two or three times, but suppose father had some spark of parental feeling left, so he induced me to return home again. The best friend I had in those days was my father's brother, Mr. Merrick, hair Dresser, Church Gate, Leicester.

When about 13 years old, nothing would satisfy my step-mother until she got me out to work; I obtained employment at Messrs. Freeman's Cigar Manufacturers, and worked there about two years, but my right hand got too heavy for making cigars, so I had to leave them.

I was sent about the town to see if I could procure work, but being lame and deformed no one would employ me; when I went home for my meals, my step-mother used to say I had not been to seek for work. I was taunted and sneered at so that I would not go home for my meals, and used to stay in the streets with an hungry belly rather than return for anything to eat, what few half-meals I did have,

I was taunted with the remark—"That's more than you have earned."

Being unable to get employment my father got me a pedlar's license to hawk the town, but being deformed, people would not come to the door to buy my wares. In consequence of my ill luck my life was again made a misery to me, so that I again ran away and went hawking on my own account, but my deformity had grown to such an extent, so that I could not move about the town without having a crowd of people gather around me. I then went into the infirmary at Leicester, where I remained for two or three years, when I had to undergo an operation on my face, having three or four ounces of flesh cut away; so thought I, I'll get my living by being exhibited about the country. Knowing Mr. Sam Torr, Gladstone Vaults, Wharf Street, Leicester, went in for Novelties, I wrote to him, he came to see me, and soon arranged matters, recommending me to Mr. Ellis, Bee-hive Inn, Nottingham, from whom I received the greatest kindness and attention.

In making my first appearance before the public, who have treated me well—in fact I may say I am as comfortable now as I was uncomfortable before. I must now bid my kind readers adieu."

The Elephant Man in the News

"THE ELEPHANT MAN."

TO THE EDITOR OF THE TIMES.

Sir,—I am authorized to ask your powerful assistance in bringing to the notice of the public the following most exceptional case. There is now in a little room off one of our attic wards a man named Joseph Merrick, aged about 27, a native of Leicester, so dreadful a sight that he is unable even to come out by daylight to the garden. He has been called "the elephant man" on account of his terrible deformity. I will not shock your readers with any detailed description of his infirmities, but only one arm is available for work.

Some 18 month ago, Mr. Treves, one of the surgeons of the London Hospital, saw him as he was exhibited in a room off the Whitechapel-road. The poor fellow was then covered by an old curtain, endeavouring to warm himself over a brick which was heated by a lamp. As soon as a sufficient number of pennies had been collected by the manager at the door, poor Merrick threw off his curtain and exhibited himself in all his deformity. He and the manager went halves in the net proceeds of this exhibition, until at last the police stopped the exhibition of his deformities as against public decency.

Unable to earn his livelihood by exhibiting himself any longer in England, he was persuaded to go over to Belgium, where he was taken in hand by an Austrian, who acted as his manager. Merrick managed in this way to save a sum of nearly £50, but the police there too kept him moving on, so that his life was a miserable and hunted one. One day, however, when the Austrian saw that the exhibition was pretty well played out, he decamped with poor Merrick's hardly-saved capital of £50, and left him alone and absolutely destitute in a foreign country. Fortunately, however, he had something to pawn, by which he raised sufficient money to pay his passage back to England, for he felt that the only friend he had in the world was Mr. Treves, of the London Hospital. He therefore, though with much difficulty, made his way there, for at every station and landing-place the curious crowd so thronged and dogged his steps that it was not an easy matter for him to get about. When he reached the London Hospital he had only the clothes in which he stood. He has been taken in by our hospital, though there is, unfortunately, no hope of his cure, and the question now arises what is to be done with him in the future.

He has the greatest horror of the workhouse, nor is it possible, indeed, to send him into any place where he could not insure privacy, since his appearance is such that all shrink from him.

The Royal Hospital for Incurables and the British Home for Incurables both decline to take him in, even if sufficient funds were forthcoming to pay for him.

The police rightly prevent his being personally exhibited again ; he cannot go out into the streets, as he is everywhere so mobbed that existence is impossible ; he cannot, in justice to others, be put in the general ward of a workhouse, and from such, even if possible, he shrinks with the greatest horror ; he ought not to be detained in our hospital (where he is occupying a private ward, and being treated with the greatest kindness—he says he has never before known in his life what quiet and rest were), since his case is incurable, and not suited, therefore, to our overcrowded general hospital ; the incurable hospitals refuse to take him in even if we paid for him in full, and the difficult question therefore remains what is to be done for him.

Terrible though his appearance is, so terrible indeed that women and nervous persons fly in terror from the sight of him, and that he is debarred from seeking to earn his livelihood in any ordinary way, yet he is superior in intelligence, can read and write, is quiet, gentle, not to say even refined in his mind. He occupies his time in the hospital by making with his one available hand little cardboard models, which he sends to the matron, doctor, and those who have been kind to him. Through all the miserable vicissitudes of his life he has carried about a painting of his mother to show that she was a decent and presentable person, and as a memorial of the only one who was kind to him in life until he came under the kind care of the nursing staff of the London Hospital and the surgeon who has befriended him.

It is a case of singular affliction brought about through no fault of himself ; he can but hope for quiet and privacy during a life which Mr. Treves assures me is not likely to be long.

Can any of your readers suggest to me some fitting place where he can be received ? And then I feel sure that, when that is found, charitable people will come forward and enable me to provide him with such accommodation. In the meantime, though it is not the proper place for such an incurable case, the little room under the roof of our hospital and out of Cotton Ward supplies him with all he wants. The Master of the Temple on Advent Sunday preached an eloquent sermon on the subject of our Master's answer to the question, " Who did sin, this man or his parents, that he was born blind ? " showing how one of the Creator's objects in permitting men to be born to a life of hopeless and miserable disability was that the works of God should be manifested in evoking the sympathy and kindly aid of those on whom such a heavy cross is not laid.

Some 76,000 patients a year pass through the doors of our hospital, but I have never before been authorized to invite public attention to any particular case, so it may well be believed that this case is exceptional.

Any communication about this should be addressed either to myself or to the secretary at the London Hospital.

I have the honour to be, Sir, yours obediently,

F. C. CARR GOMM, Chairman London Hospital.
November 30.

The Times, December 4, 1886.

"THE ELEPHANT MAN."

TO THE EDITOR OF THE TIMES.

Sir,—In a letter which you were kind enough to insert some weeks back about Joseph Merrick, who had formerly been exhibited under the name of " the Elephant Man " I asked whether any one could suggest a fitting home where he could be received, adding that I felt sure when such a home was found charitable people would come forward and enable me to place him therein. The letter interested many, and I received numerous kind answers from all parts of the country, and had my appeal been directly for money I am convinced abundance would have speedily been sent to me.

The practical result of the correspondence is that no home is to be found so suitable to his needs as the hospital, and we now feel ourselves justified in keeping him with us ; and although a general hospital supported by voluntary contributions is strictly for curative purposes where each occupied bed represents an outlay little short of £70 per annum, our committee have decided under the peculiar circumstances to set apart a small room where the poor fellow not only secures that privacy which is so essential to his comfort, but also is supplied with all that can possibly alleviate his sad condition, such as baths, good nursing, and medical supervision.

This is in accordance with the wishes expressed by most of the contributors, and Merrick himself, naturally enough, much prefers remaining where he has found so much sympathy and comfort.

His generous supporters will be glad to hear of our decision, and Merrick has desired me to convey to them his most grateful thanks, and to say that he is deeply sensible of their kindness and that he has never had so happy and peaceful a Christmas time as he has had now. He is newly clothed and well supplied with books and papers, while the kind care of the sister and nurses, with visits from the chaplain and others, relieves the monotony of his existence. One lady has most thoughtfully engaged to provide for his being taught basket-making, to give him some definite occupation, and I hope at once to start this work.

If he leaves us, and he is of course a free agent, I shall now be able to provide for his being properly taken care of by an uncle at Leicester, who is too poor a man to take him in unless means were given him, but there can be no question that he is far better off with us than he could possibly be outside, and this is his own feeling.

As I have personally replied to each one who has written except, of course, anonymous contributors, I have not thought it necessary to publish any list, but I have received and hold in trust sufficient to enable me to provide for the poor fellow's comfort for some four or five years to come, and if more should then be required, I will ask for it.

As many have desired to know particulars of this unique case, I would add that some details are given, with illustrations, in the *British Medical Journal* of the 11th ultimo, one of our objects, however, is to prevent his deformity being made anything of a show, except for purely scientific purposes, and the hospital officials have instructions to secure for him as far as possible immunity from the gaze of the curious.

I have the honour to be, Sir, yours obediently,
F. C. CARR-GOMM, Chairman of the London Hospital.
London Hospital, Whitechapel-road, E., Jan. 3.

The Times, January 5, 1887.

THE ELEPHANT MAN.

A Strangely Deformed Human Being Who Is Interesting Medical Men.

[London Correspondent Philadelphia Telegraph.]

I have been hearing a good deal lately about the elephant man, as he is commonly called, for he has been creating much interest in medical circles, and even in general society. This poor creature, whose name is John Derrick, is suffering from a variety of complex diseases, which give him the appearance of a most extraordinary monster. His skin hangs in great folds on his disproportioned body; he has an immense bony enlargement of the head, which makes it so much too large for his body that he is never allowed to lie down, but has to sleep with it on his knees, and his mouth is so extraordinarily displaced that he can not drink without jerking his head right back. One leg is three or four times larger than the other, and in the hands there is a similar disparity. His life, though he is only twenty-eight, has been a very curious one, a large portion of it having been spent in traveling shows in various countries. On the last occasion he was persuaded to accompany a man to Belgium, but when he got there this heartless wretch borrowed all his savings and left him penniless and helpless in a strange country. With great difficulty he managed to get to London, for such is the horror of his aspect that he is not allowed to walk in the streets, and the steamers at first refused to take him. His troubles are now to a great extent over, for funds have been collected to maintain him. Derrick is most grateful for any kindness shown him, and is always delighted to see any visitors. The Prince and Princess of Wales, when they went over the London Hospital, they spent a few minutes with him, which gave him very great pleasure, and for several days he could talk and think of nothing else.

A touching incident is told of how a lady went to see him when he was first at the hospital, and on her shaking hands with him he burst into tears. With great difficulty he was persuaded to tell the cause of his distress, but at last he confessed that never before had a woman shaken hands with him; they had usually screamed with horror at his approach. Derrick is wonderfully contented, and manages to amuse himself by making models of buildings and ships very cleverly out of cardboard, wood, cork, etc. His other favorite occupation is reading sensational novels of the most thrilling and bloodthirsty type. Once he has even been taken to the theater, in accordance with the wish of his heart. The royal box at Drury Lane was given him for an afternoon performance; he used the Queen's private entrance, and few present were aware that the uncouth man of whom they had heard was enjoying the pantomime with them. Derrick was entranced by all he saw, and no wonder, for it must have seemed like a dream to the poor creature who had seen nothing of the bright side of life.

The care and treatment he receives are gradually strengthening him, though he can never hope to recover in the least from the horrible disease with which he is afflicted, and which, to a certain extent, he has had from his birth. He quite realizes the interest which science takes in his case, and one day remarked to a doctor who was visiting him: "Do you know, sir, it often strikes me that when I die I shan't be buried." The thought, however, of being preserved after death as a curious "specimen" did not seem in any way to give him pain. As a proof of the interest which is taken in his case, I may mention that on hearing he had a great desire to possess a watch Lady Dorothy Neville got up a subscription to provide him with one. Several royalties, including H. R. H. the Prince of Wales, and H. R. H. the Duke of Cambridge, gave donations, and over £100 was collected, which was spent in buying him a most beautiful chronometer.

Louisville Courier Journal, March 23, 1888.

DEATH OF "THE ELEPHANT MAN."

An inquest on the body of Joseph Merrick, better known as the "Elephant Man," was held yesterday at the London Hospital by Mr. Baxter. Charles Merrick, of Church-gate, Leicester, a hairdresser, identified the body as that of his nephew. The deceased was 29 years of age, and had followed no occupation. From birth he had been deformed, but he got much worse of late. He had been in the hospital four or five years. His parents were in no way afflicted, and the father, an engine driver, is alive now. Mr. Ashe, house surgeon, said he was called to the deceased at 3 30 p.m. on Friday, and found him dead. It was expected that he would die suddenly. There were no marks of violence, and the death was quite natural. The man had great overgrowth of the skin and bone, but he did not complain of anything. Witness believed that the exact cause of death was asphyxia, the back of his head being greatly deformed, and while the patient was taking a natural sleep the weight of the head overcame him, and so suffocated him. The coroner said that the man had been sent round the shows as a curiosity, and when death took place it was decided as a matter of prudence to hold this inquest. Mr. Hodges, another house surgeon, stated that on Friday last he went to visit the deceased, and found him lying across the bed dead. He was in a ward specially set apart for him. Witness did not touch him. Nurse Ireland, of the Blizzard Ward, said the deceased was in her charge. She saw him on Friday morning, when he appeared in his usual health. His midday meal was taken in to him, but he did not touch it. The coroner, in summing up, said there could be no doubt that death was quite in accordance with the theory put forward by the doctor. The jury accepted this view, and returned a verdict to the effect that death was due to suffocation from the weight of the head pressing on the windpipe.

The Times, April 16, 1890.

An Image Gallery of Joseph Merrick

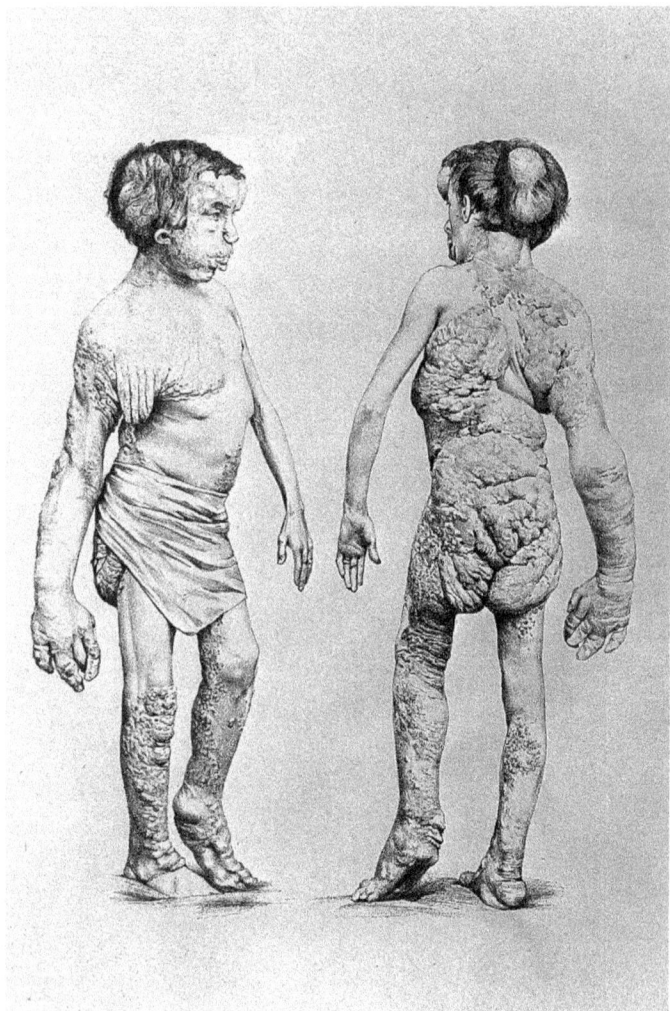

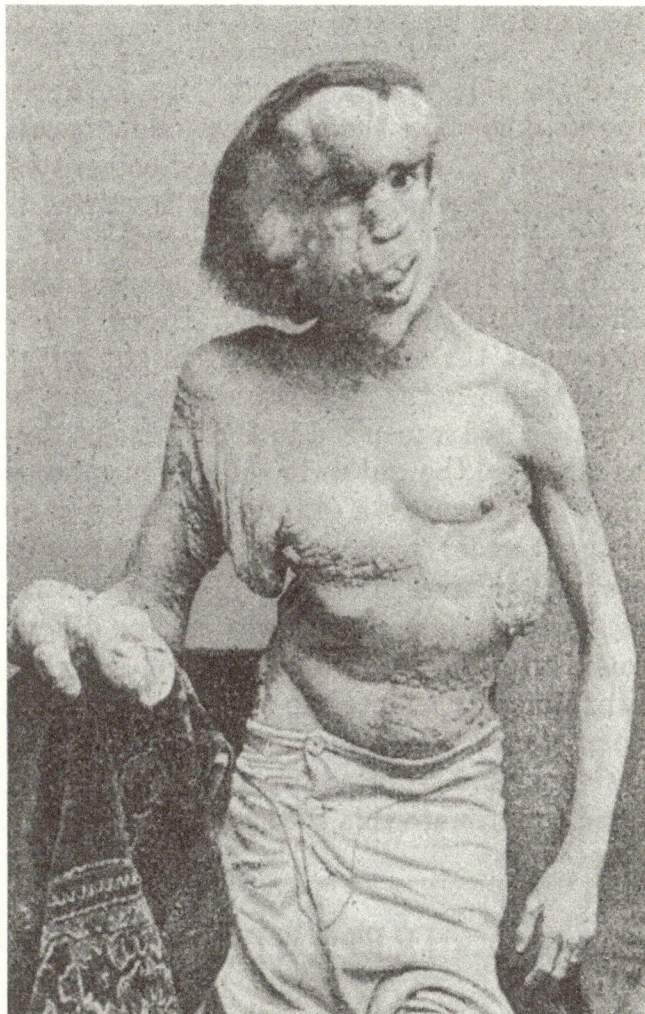

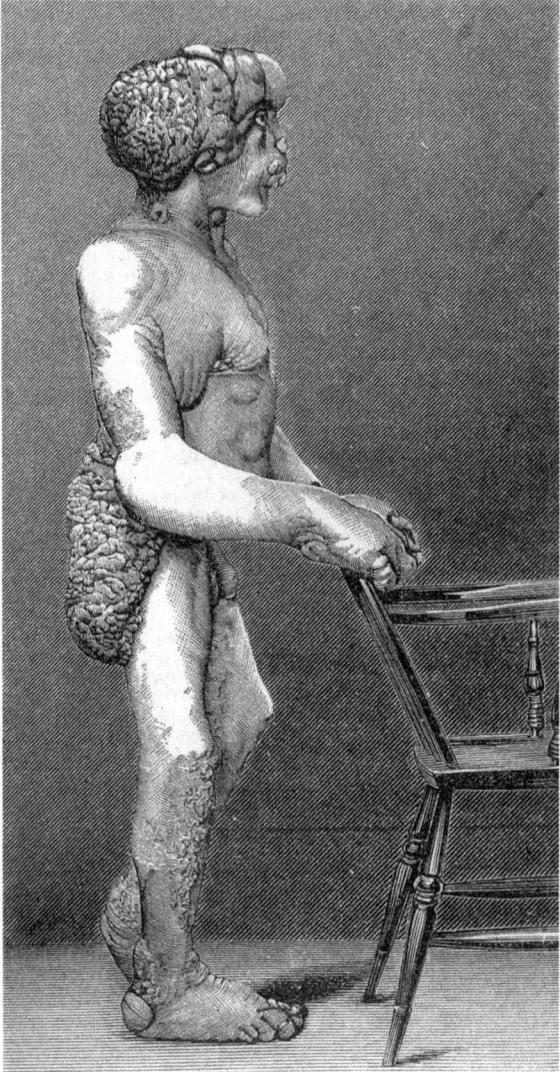

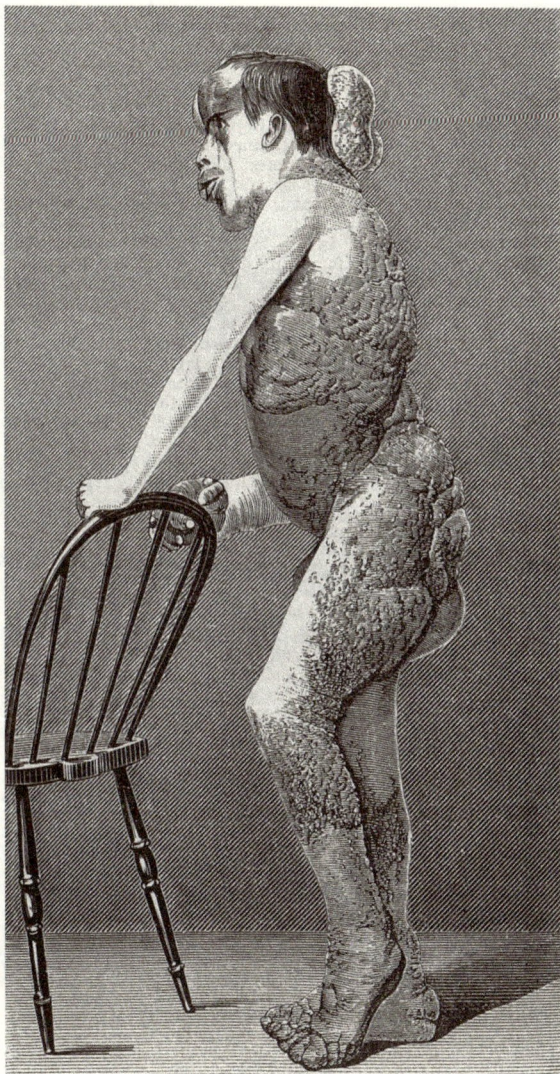

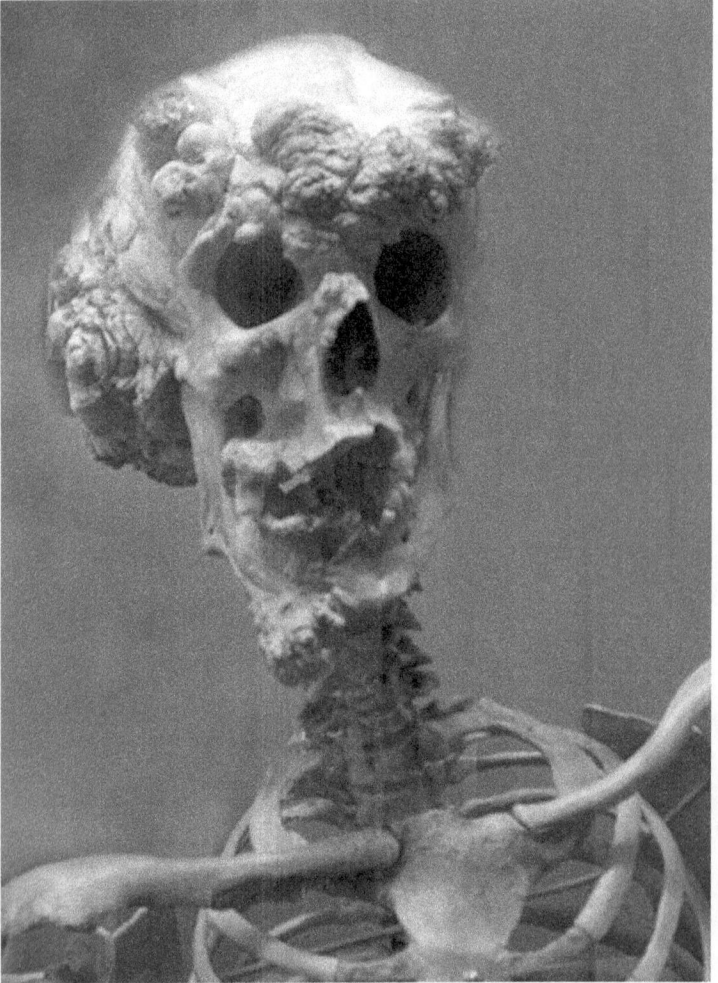

Replica of Joseph Merrick's skeleton at the Royal London Hospital.

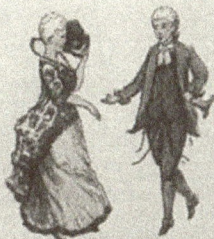

Dear Miss Maturin

Many thanks indeed for the grouse, and the book, you so kindly sent me, the grouse were splendid I saw Mr Treves on Sunday He said I was to give his best respects to you With much Gratitude I am Yours Truly

Joseph Merrick.

London Hospital

Whitechapel

Letter to Leila Maturin, a widow from the Isle of Islay who greeted Merrick and shook his hand, offering him a moment of humanity few others had.

ALSO FROM
CURIOUS PUBLICATIONS

curiouspublications.com